The
Knowles
Method of Breath
Training

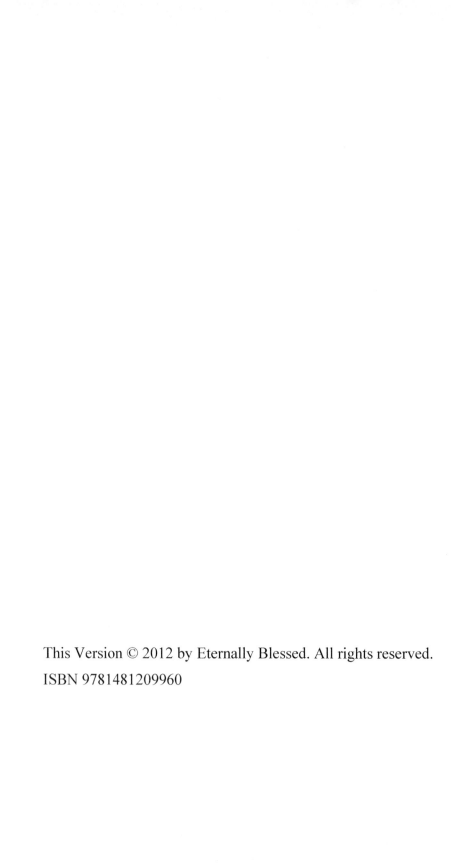

ISBN 9781481209960

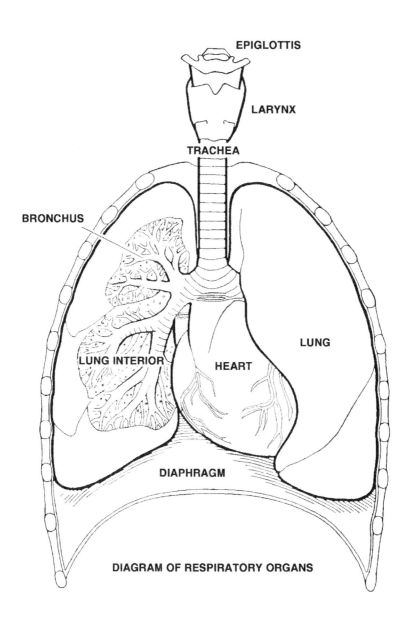

EPIGLOTTIS

LARYNX

TRACHEA

BRONCHUS

LUNG

LUNG INTERIOR

HEART

DIAPHRAGM

DIAGRAM OF RESPIRATORY ORGANS

Foreword

In recent years, numerous clinical studies have demonstrated the physical and mental benefits resulting from a regular regimen of breathing techniques. Tremendous improvements to overall health and well- being have been directly proven to issue from consistently followed, proper breathing exercises.

- Studies reported in the *American Journal of Hypertension*, provide proof that such exercises markedly reduce high blood pressure.

- A randomized, controlled trial study conducted at the University of California, San Francisco cites, "Patients suffering from chronic low back pain (CLBP) are often unsatisfied with conventional medical care and seek alternative therapies. Patients suffering from CLBP improved significantly with breath therapy. Changes in standard low back pain measures of pain and disability were comparable to those resulting from high quality, extended physical therapy."

- A recent clinical trial published in the *American Journal of Gastroenterology* showed that "...deep breathing exercises could actually prevent heartburn and relieve existing symptoms."

- *The International Journal of Neuroscience* states that numerous clinical studies attest to the benefits of deep breathing exercises improve mental performance.

- Furthermore, the US Department of Health and Human Services extensively reviewed clinical studies carried out by numerous organizations throughout the world over a period of several years. The findings of their report corroborate the anecdotal evidence that breathing techniques significantly reduce stress, enhance energy and vitality, improve mental health and function, reduce high blood pressure, improved pulmonary function, and provided relief to asthma sufferers.

Long before all of these clinical studies were conducted, William P. Knowles shared the testimony of hundreds of people whose lives were changed and health restored as a result of the method of breath training he developed. Having overcome serious health issues himself through the practice of breathing exercises, he developed a proven method of breath training. He began teaching that method to dramatically improve the health and well-being of people, and during World War II the British Armed Forces employed Knowles to teach the same techniques to the Royal Air Force. Throughout his life, Knowles helped thousands of people through his individual instruction and publications.

In the latter part of the 20th century, many more thousands of people were introduced to *The Knowles Method of Breath Training* through the efforts of Victor Paul Wierwille. The Reverend Dr. Victor Paul Wierwille founded and presided over a worldwide Biblical research, teaching, and fellowship ministry. As a minister, VP Wierwille was concerned about helping people to be their best physically and mentally, as well as spiritually. In addition to the extensive curriculum of Biblical studies, students at his campuses received instruction in such beneficial, practical matters as healthy eating and all aspects of physical fitness. Dr. Wierwille was greatly impressed with Knowles' work, and he highly encouraged his students to study and practice the techniques.

Today, many enthusiastic practitioners of the Knowles method continue to enjoy the benefits of health and well-being gained through breath training. When faithfully carried out, the simple method taught in this book will provide the reader with energy, vitality, and renewed strength to resist and fight disease.

The objects of this course are to enhance the qualities of your body and mind, through correct breathing, to give you added resistance to illness, and to help overcome illness if it strikes. Its highest aim is to have you prove to yourself by results that your Body, Mind and even Spirit depend equally for their health, harmony and development upon your breathing.

If "Breath of Life"—and who would deny it?—then to be conscious of Life we must be conscious of Breath. We cannot help breathing so long as we live, and most people imagine that everyone breathes correctly by nature: therefore why need we concern ourselves about it? But this idea, as you will presently realize, is not true. The changing habits of civilized man, especially *urban* man, have altered Nature's techniques and often reduced their efficiency. This is particularly true of breathing. But there is a breathing technique which can make us far fitter men and women. Indeed, breath properly used gives more than physical fitness; it calms the mind and even helps morale.

Have you ever stopped to think what is the most important thing in life to you? Is it money, love, friendship, philosophy, art, science, or possessions of some kind? All these things have their value; but *the* most important factor for each one of us is life itself; and in life it is breath which is the most immediate vital agent. What would all the other things be worth if breath suddenly failed us?

There is an old Persian proverb which says: "Life is the pause between one breath and another", which focuses our attention on that something we call breath, upon which all life depends. It is one thing to say glibly, "Breath is Life"; it is quite another matter to *realize* it. We may understand intellectually that something exists, and how it exists; but until it becomes *vital* and *real*—a living reality in our lives—we do not realize it. I hope to make breathing a vital reality to you.

The main question which must be faced and answered is: How can you make breath give you a mind and a body which can be relied upon to do all that you demand of them, subject to the general rules of health? The answer—the only answer—is: by the constant practice of correct breathing which will give you a continual supply of energy, mental power and general well-being.

How to improve your lungs

As any physiologist would agree, most people use only a portion of their lung capacity. The first step, then, must be to increase the use of the lungs in order that better health, better resistance to disease, stronger nerves and more vitality may result from the breathing IN of more life—giving oxygen, and the breathing OUT of the waste air with its load of poisons that creates fatigue and ill-health.

Another fact is that the human brain is never used to capacity; and indeed much of it is probably never developed. Opinions differ as to the capacity of the brain, and reasons for the shortcomings often shown in its use. There is a strong probability that many human brains lack their fully required supply of oxygen.

The question remains: *How* can the activity of the lungs be increased? How can they be made to do a better job?

What you must do at first

First, attention must be given to bodily POSTURE. You will get full benefit from the exercises given in this course only if you practice them in the right posture. Relaxation is also important and will be dealt with in the next lesson, but posture matters most at the beginning.

Have you ever seen the Egyptian royal statues in the British museum, or illustrations of them? The figures were carved some thousands of years ago: they all sit with straight backs, their hands on their thighs. Was this bodily pose intentional? Certainly the Egyptian sculptors were masters of sculptural technique and showed that they observed both nature and their masters with great accuracy. It is obvious from both sculpture and paintings that physical uprightness was an everyday feature of their lives, and a truly royal posture. From the health standpoint, they were absolutely correct. So we want to get the upright pose of the Egyptian statues in our posture—with one small difference: this difference is in the proudly-carried head. Not being forced to hold the head royally high, we should drop the head slightly down so that the neck and throat are quite relaxed.

Choose a hard chair. If it is too high, place a book or rest under your feet. If it is too low, place a book on the chair to raise the seat. Sit down on this chair, bolt upright, and, as a separate movement, draw the shoulder blades together, while keeping the chest firm by pressing the shoulders gently back and slightly down.

Keeping the shoulders in this position is most important throughout all the exercises

The simplest way to do this is to tuck your elbows into your side, raising your hands horizontally. Then, keeping the hands in the horizontal position, (and with elbows still hugging the side) draw back the arms as far as they will go without straining. Then lower the hands on to the thighs. By so doing, you will have brought the shoulder blades together. In this position you cannot drop the chest nor distend the abdomen, and you will give free play to the "breathing" muscles of the diaphragm and chest.

The feet should be placed a little apart and pointing slightly outwards: the knees should be slightly apart. The spine should be held away from the back of the chair. The body should lean slightly forward. The head should be slightly bent.

If you feel more comfortable standing up, keep the shoulders back and down (as in the sitting posture), and the arms hanging loosely at the sides. The feet should be placed a little way apart, and pointing a little outwards.

Now when you are ready, relax the facial muscles thoroughly. Take your time in doing this. "Think into" each feature of your face; feel each feature gently relaxing. Then rest the tongue gently against the inside of the lower teeth. Keep the teeth slightly apart and close the lips. This will ease the nasal cavities and sinuses, so that full advantage of the breath can be taken. Now we are ready to breathe.

ALWAYS BREATHE IN AND OUT THROUGH THE NOSE because the nose:
    a.   warms the incoming air;
    b.   cleans it;
    c.   moistens it;
    d.   kills germs.

In order to ensure that the in-breathed air enters the lung in the most favourable state, the nose supplies some vital services. Tissues inside the nose, warmed by a particularly rich blood supply, act like an efficient radiator, and as the air passes over them it is automatically warmed before being warmed still more in the windpipe. Also inside the nose is a forest of minute hairs (cilia), which trap much of the grit, dust and other "debris" which we are forced to take in when we breathe. More particles of "debris" are trapped by the sticky surface of the mucous which is secreted by glands in the nose. Both mucous and tears (which constantly bathe the eyes and find their way into the nose through ducts) serve to moisten the air as it comes into the body, so that it does not lend to dry the windpipe, and bronchi as it goes down. Finally, an enzyme named *lysozyme* is present in the mucous and tears, and this enzyme is one of the most powerful bacteria killers known.

Incidentally, the microscopic hairs (cilia) mentioned above, are also to be found lining the surfaces of the windpipe, bronchi and bronchioles. Their function and operation are remarkable because they continually beat (or flail as it is called) in *one direction,* and that direction is *upwards.* So that there is a perpetually operating scavenging service provided to clean the air passages, the "refuse" of which is fed up the windpipe, into the esophagus, and harmlessly down into the stomach.

Our ordinary everyday breathing causes a tide of air (called the "tidal" air) to pass in and out of the lungs. The amount that flows in and out in this tide from actual breathing is small compared with the amount of air which remains in the lungs all the time, which is called "residual" air. Therefore, to start our breathing exercises properly, the lungs should be cleansed of as much impure air as possible. This is accomplished by a Cleansing Breath, which we take as follows:

EXERCISE 1. The Cleansing Breath. First, breathe *in* as deeply and comfortably as you can. Then breath *out* and in, *out* and in, *out* and in, to the rhythm of sawing wood, where the out-breath is the working stroke and the in-breath is the pull-back recovery stroke, always breathing o u t more breath forcibly than you breathe in. Go on breathing *out* and in, *out* and in, in this way until you cannot breathe out any more. Then purse your l i p s and blow out. You will find you can still puff out quite a good b i t of air. Pause a second. Then let the long satisfying in-breath sweep into your lungs automatically. Then start again, and do this exercise three or four times.

It is important that you should keep your chest out and your shoulders back, in the posture I have described. This posture ensures that all the muscles engaged in breathing especially the intercostal muscles in the chest, can move more freely and without strain, and hence operate to expand the lungs as much as possible.

EXERCISE 2. Slow and Deep Breathing. Keeping the upright posture as already described, start to fill your lungs to their fullest capacity, but *do not strain* in any way. Breathe IN while you count four seconds silently. Pause a second. Then, *without lowering the chest,* breathe OUT to the count of four seconds. Again pause. Next breathe in to a count of five seconds. Pause a second. Breathe out to the count of five. Pause. Another breath in to the count of six—and out. Finally, breathe in to the count of seven and out again. Another breath to six counts, then five, and finishing with four counts.

4

A good way of counting the seconds of in- and out- breathing is to say silently to yourself: *"one* and *two* and *three* and *four* and *pause* and *one* and *two* and *three* and *four* and *pause* (etc.)", the insertion of the "ands" gives an easy rhythm to the counts. So now, to repeat:

Breathe IN	Breathe OUT
to a count of 4 seconds	to a count of 4 seconds
" " 5 "	" " 5 "
" " 6 "	" " 6 "
" " 7 "	" " 7 "
" " 6 "	" " 6 "
" " 5 "	" " 5 "
" " 4 "	" " 4 "

This exercise takes approximately 1½ minutes; it should be repeated at each period of exercising.

In the exercise I have just described, an even breath-rhythm should be kept up. When breathing IN to the count of 1 to 4, the breathing OUT must also be to the count of 1 to 4, with the lungs being filled and emptied in each motion of 4 counts. The lungs must always be filled and emptied to the utmost (without strain) whether this takes place in breaths of 4 or 7 counts. Care should be taken to pause for one second at the end of both the inward and the outward actions. The pause after breathing IN allows time for the air which is rushing into the lungs to mix thoroughly with, and freshen up with new oxygen, the residual air already in the millions of minute air-tubes and sacs. Then the wafer-thin walls of these air-sacs (alveoli) can give the blood a new supply of oxygen and receive back from the blood its waste carbon dioxide. The pause after breathing OUT allows the impure air carrying the waste carbon dioxide to get clear of the lungs before the next in-breath.

Breath as purifier

Every sense and every function of the human body ultimately depends upon the purifying process of breath. Therefore, the circulation of the blood, the action of the nerves and the secretions of the glands are benefited by the increased intake of breath and the higher percentage of oxygen. Most people breathe '"unconsciously" to a rhythm of from 14 to 18 breath-cycles (in- and out-breaths) per minute, or a breath of 3-4 seconds in, and 3-4 seconds out. This has been called the "Mother Breath" because it is the breath passed on by the mother during the period when she breathed *for* the child. A child does not use its own lungs until it has been born. It then continues the rhythm of the mother's breathing.

Our first main action, apart from the cleansing breath, has been to expand the lungs (without strain) by increasing their capacity. Our first exercise commences where the mother's breath left off—a new breath of four seconds in and four seconds out (with a second's pause at top and bottom) being taken. The object is to train the nervous system to get used to and accept the *idea* of a longer and deeper breath. Once this idea is accepted, it will soon be obeyed automatically. Therefore the exercise should be practiced daily. 3 times a day. The records of my students have shown that the habit of longer and deeper breathing comes after some three weeks' exercise; there is a better nerve action in the brain, and improved glandular flow upon which all mental development ultimately depends.

Each exercise in slower and deeper breathing should be continued for approximately 3 minutes to ensure proper oxygenation of the blood.

The student should always mentally follow the passage of breath through the nose, the air-tubes and the lungs, keeping in mind its power to bring cleansing and life-giving oxygen to the blood system. This helps to bring about the *realization* I mentioned previously.

Points to remember:

Observe the posture instructions carefully. Remember that the wall of the chest should be held high and firm both during breathing IN (*Inhaling*) and breathing OUT (*Exhaling*): before you have finished this course, you should find yourself doing this automatically. Remember also to fill the lungs as completely as possible, whatever rhythm or count you are breathing to, and to breathe out as completely as you can: but don't strain or strive: take it easy. Breathe in and out *through the nose.* Be careful not to arch the back when bringing the shoulder blades together. The closeness of the shoulder blades is the most important point throughout the exercise. Finally, remember that the key to success lies in regular practice.

N.B. The exercises should be practiced for at least THREE MINUTES at a time, and at least THREE TIMES DAILY; oftener if you wish.

Exercise 1 and 2 are simple, but they form the foundation upon which the science of correct breathing is based. Later you will learn how to:

(*a*) Increase the whole depth of breathing, and strengthen your diaphragm and intercostal muscles for breathing OUT slowly.

(*b*) Strengthen your diaphragm and intercostal muscles for breathing IN, thus allowing you to inhale a greater amount of air, and hence a greater supply of oxygen, allowing the nerves to relax, and resulting in a calmer state of mind.

(*c*) Retain the oxygen after increased inhalation to strengthen and tone up the mental controls, improving memory and the power of concentration.

(*d*) Apply the power of correct breathing to Digestion, Assimilation and Excretion.

(*e*) Control your own vital forces.

The time it will take you to learn to breathe correctly will depend upon the regularity of your practice.

How to Resist Disease and Ill Health

Postal Course: **LESSON TWO**

Before proceeding with this Second Lesson, remember the two important instructions set out in Lesson One. i.e. to adopt the correct **posture**, but to do so in a **relaxed way**. It is also useful to be able to concentrate your attention at will, especially to concentrate it positively and constructively. One way to do this is to focus your eyes comfortably on some small object before you and give yourself the thought that you are going to breathe correctly and exercise regularly. If Exercise Two (the four-second breath) has been conscientiously practiced for two weeks, three minutes at a time, three times a day, you are ready for the next step. Continue to practice Exercise One (the cleansing breath) before you start, but discontinue Exercise Two in favour of the following exercise.

EXERCISE 3. The Seven-second Breath. Sit down or stand up as before, carefully following the instructions for posture given in Lesson One. Take the cleansing breath as before. Then breathe OUT without lowering the chest. Now breathe IN to the count of seven seconds; pause a second; then breathe OUT seven seconds. Pause a second and repeat. Do this in-and-out breath cycle twelve times.

This exercise can be performed sitting, standing or lying down. When walking, step off with the left foot and count four steps as you breathe in; pause for one step; breathe out to a count of four steps, again pause for a step and repeat. Remember, twelve times is all that is necessary to oxygenate the blood thoroughly as it flows round the body first as good fresh "arterial" blood through the arteries, and then back through the veins, as stale "venous" blood to the heart.

This exercise may well be termed the "corner-stone" of the science of breathing. When it is carried out consistently (three times daily), Nature will respond to your effort, and a new rhythm will be set up in the nerves and bloodstream, giving you new vitality and energy. Having got a rhythmic breath and learned how to direct the breathing consciously, you will be able to breathe without strain.

Lengthening the outward breath (exhalation)

Most people accumulate an excess of carbon dioxide (CO_2) in the blood every three to five hours. This is also one of the reasons why we yawn. It is Nature prompting us to breathe OUT more thoroughly—the way to get rid of the waste carbon we do not need. Too much carbon causes carbonated blood in which disease germs breed freely. In fact, science uses carbonated blood for bacterial culture, and epidemics spread rapidly when contagious disease finds the blood overloaded with carbon. Lengthening the outward breath rids the blood of this excess, and increases resistance to disease. Most of us breathe IN to better effect than we breathe OUT, and to increase the outward breath is therefore not an easy exercise. But breathing OUT as fully as possible is one of the vital secrets of good breathing. Once again I must remind you of the following points:

POSTURE – The chest wall should be kept firm: if you keep the shoulder blades together you cannot drop the chest. But remember—no tension, just poise.

CONCENTRATION – Without this, you will not be able to maintain the position of the chest wall.

RELAXATION – This will not only keep your posture and movements easy or calm, but also enable the diaphragm to recoil smoothly and easily before being pulled down for the next in-breath.

EXERCISE 4. Lengthening the Outward Breath. The two main purposes of this exercise are to rid the blood of excess carbon dioxide, and to strengthen the out-breathing muscles. Therefore the **breathing OUT will be 3 times longer than the breathing IN,** commencing to a count of 4 seconds, and getting progressively longer.

Care must be taken (1) to keep the shoulder blades close together; (2) not to breathe out too quickly—just a gentle steady exhalation—pausing for a second at the end of the breath; (3) to pause for a second at the end of the inward breath. These pauses in the exercises are very important.

So take up your posture either sitting or standing, remembering to bring the shoulder blades back and slightly down so that the elbows touch the sides of the body. Remember to drop the chin slightly; relax the face muscles and neck; place the tongue against the inside of the lower teeth; keep the teeth a little apart and the lips closed. Next, take the cleansing breath—about the rhythm of sawing wood—Out-in, out-in, out-in, until you can't comfortably go on: then puff out the air you will find still available; pause; and breathe in slowly; then breathe out slowly and fully. Be sure you do not tense up; keep as relaxed as possible at all times.

NOW FOR THE EXERCISE: Breathe **IN** to the count of **4**, taking care to fill the lungs completely, right up to the top: pause a second, then (keeping the chest-wall firm) breathe slowly **OUT** to a count of twelve: i.e. **one** and **two** and **three** and **four** and **five** and **six** and **seven** and **eight** and **nine** and **ten** and **eleven** and **twelve** and pause (now breathe **IN**) and **one** and **two** and **three** and **four** and **five** and pause (now breathe **OUT**) and **one** and **two** and **three** and **four** and **five** and **six** and **seven** and **eight** and **nine** and **ten** and **eleven** and **twelve** and **thirteen** and **fourteen** and **fifteen** and pause (now breathe **IN**) and **one** and **two** and **three** and **four** and **five** and **six** and pause (now breathe **OUT**) and **one** and **two** and **three** and **four** and **five** and **six** and **seven** and **eight** and **nine** and **ten** and **eleven** and **twelve** and **thirteen** and **fourteen** and **fifteen** and **sixteen** and **seventeen** and **eighteen** and pause (now breathe **IN**) and **one** and **two** and **three** and **four** and **five** and **six** and **seven** and pause (now breathe **OUT**) and **one** and **two** and **three** and **four** and **five** and **six** and **seven** and **eight** and **nine** and **ten** and **eleven** and **twelve** and **thirteen** and **fourteen** and **fifteen** and **sixteen** and **seventeen** and **eighteen** and **nineteen** and **twenty**. Repeat this last count three times.

More about relaxation

Many a book could be written about Relaxation. It is a fairly simple matter consciously to relax the muscles known as the "striped" (striated) muscles through our control of the central nervous system, but it is much more difficult to relax the "smooth" (unstriated) muscles over which we can exercise no direct control. Many nervous troubles begin with tension in the sympathetic (autonomous) nervous system controlling the smooth muscles. We are often not aware of this tension, and correct breathing is one of the best remedies.

So you have to learn to breathe **OUT** until you reach the point where you utterly resign the physical body to the thought of complete relaxation.

Do not think that you cannot relax because you are sitting erect with a straight spine, or standing. The secret of relaxation is to **poise** the body, not to allow it to "slump" when sitting, or "slouch" when standing. With a little practice, you will find yourself able to sit in the upright posture without fatigue for hours at a time, or—for shorter periods—to stand without fatigue.

Reminder about the lungs

The main points to remember are that in normal breathing, the dome-like floor of muscle called the diaphragm, and the intercostal muscles of the ribs, move down and out, respectively, and enlarge the lungs, thus enlarging the air-tubes in the lungs. This creates a partial vacuum in the tubes, and causes us to breathe in air which rushes down to fill up the partial vacuum. This brings new air (and hence new oxygen) to mix with and freshen the residual air already there, and so give the terminal air-sacs new oxygen to pass on to the blood. The recoil of the diaphragm upward, and of the ribs downward and inward, returns the lungs to their normal size, and expel the surplus air including the unwanted carbon dioxide, into the atmosphere.

I must repeat that one of the most vital aims of correct breathing is to aerate the tops (apices) and lower outer portions of the lungs properly. In many people, these areas are almost stagnant—and become a breeding ground for germs, owing to the poor movement of the diaphragm not exerting a proper stretch throughout the lungs. With the chest-wall held well out to give the lungs freer play, and the slow deep breathing, you will soon be aerating the stagnant parts of your lungs fully, and really feeling the benefit. You will also be resisting disease better, and combating it better if it comes.

Relief from catarrh

Even at this early stage of the course, marked relief is often experienced by very many students from the distressing symptoms of chronic catarrh. This is a direct result of training the lungs to fuller action.

N.B. You should now be doing the following exercises **at least** three times a day –

Exercise 1 (the cleansing breath).

Exercise 3 (the seven in and seven out).

Exercise 4 (the progressive longer breaths).

Breathing Correctly Strengthens the Nerves

Postal Course: **LESSON THREE**

Important questions

Have you mastered the technique of RELAXATION? Can you practice the preceding lessons without any effort or strain? This relaxation should become a part of your life, an unconscious attitude of mind and body which must be attained if you are going to receive maximum benefit from the course. If you don't think you are relaxing sufficiently, give extra practice or attention to it. The increased sense of well-being will soon be evident.

In all breathing exercises, remember that you prepare for exercise by first expelling as much air as possible from the lungs; by taking the cleansing breath as described in Lesson One, or an alternative cleansing breath which you may find more effective and which I will give you now. First take in a steady full breath through the nose to fill out the lungs. Then place your tongue gently against the inside of the lower teeth, and exhale through your mouth in a silent whistle, as slow as you can, until you can blow out no more. Pause. Then breathe slowly and fully IN. You will get a wonderful sensation of elation with this cleansing breath after you have learned to lengthen your out-breathing.

Remember also that all other thoughts are to be banished from your mind. No matter how excited, nervous, tired, dull or preoccupied you may be, make an effort of imagination to think only of your breathing when you are practicing each exercise. Remember what the great Frenchman Coue said: that the imagination is far stronger than the will. Make a vivid image of what you desire to do; then you will do it much more easily. The body will feel exhilarated by more normal circulation of the blood and both mind and body will be calmed and strengthened by the better control of your breath.

Exercise 5 which I will describe in this lesson is one of the most important of the series, and can be relied upon to restore the energy of body and mind quickly. By concentration on complete relaxation, the nervous system is released from sub-conscious tension, and the nerves of the autonomous (sympathetic) system are stimulated to better action. This is an important healing exercise because many ailments have their cause in the sympathetic nervous system, where tension can so easily arise, though we are often not aware of it.

Developing your lengthened breath

Each of us inherits the "Mother Breath" of approximately 3

12

seconds duration IN and 3 seconds OUT. We breathe thus unconsciously from birth. But as you have already learned, a longer breath is needed to properly replenish and fill our lungs. Our development is, therefore, literally limited by shortness of breath, while the lengthened breath brings physical, mental and spiritual forces, which are latent in every one of us, into action.

The lengthened breath needs a 7-second rhythm for its foundation. In Exercise 3 you learned how to lengthen the OUTward breath to 7 seconds. Exercise 5 will now strengthen your IN breathing muscles so that you will be able to form the habit of breathing more fully than the usual 3-second rhythm.

Body, mind and spirit

I don't expect many students to follow me or believe at first in what I am going to say. But I can assure them they will come to understand my meaning as they progress with this course. There is in all of us—or there seems to be—a unifying principle of life; a force which, when working properly in us, tends to encompass and control us, unify the diverse parts of ourselves, and gives us a sense of unity and purpose greater and higher than the mere satisfactory functioning of our minds and bodies. All beings, as the Gestalt psychologists have reminded us, are greater than the sum of their parts. Human beings are no exception. The total unified man or woman is something more than a well-functioning animal. He or she has an added stature, a stature of the spirit. We are, at our finest, spiritual beings as well as human beings. The spiritual being, the human being who has transcended purely animal nature, is the unified human being. Once one realizes this, an all-embracing force will take charge and direct the whole man or woman in body, mind and spirit. The key is, of course, religion which each student must come to for him or herself in one of its many forms. But the way of the spirit, contemplative and active, is greatly aided by the calmness and serenity of mind which the mystery of breath can help bring about. Students who seek for truth in the realm of spirit have a powerful ally in the mastery of breath.

EXCERCISE 5. Strengthening the IN-breathing Muscles. Take your seat, with all your usual care about posture. Then, when thoroughly relaxed, take a full breath **IN**, not forced, but easily. At the top of the inward breath, begin to breathe **OUT**, in a series of short breaths through the nostrils exactly like a puffing locomotive. Mentally you say **OUT**, out, out, out, until you feel you cannot breathe out any more without using strain; then pucker the lips and whistle out the remaining breath—you will find there is still some left! When the whistle dies away, keep the chest still firmly poised, hold the breath out, and arrest all movement. Remain quiet while you count 10 seconds. Then, do not gasp for breath but gently breathe **IN**—a full, deep breath. Do not move the shoulders (the tendency will be to raise them as you reach the top of the **IN**ward breath). Pause a second and again breathe **OUT** short breaths until you feel the whistle will complete the out-going breath; then hold the breath and count 15 seconds. Then repeat the slow **IN**-breath.

Control the increasing rush of your incoming breath: let it fully, yet easily, inflate the lungs. Pause a second as before and breathe **OUT**, out, out, out, out, out, out, out, out; whistle, hold the breath; keep poised and count 20 seconds. Bring the mind to bear on what you are doing so that, while you are determined, you concentrate on relaxing the body more and more, still keeping the upright posture. Then gently breathe **IN**—a full, free inhalation in which you feel the full force of the new power and capacity of your breath.

Remember, the key to posture is keeping the shoulder blades in position. This holds the chest in the correct posture without the need of any strain, and allows the intercostal muscles to raise and enlarge the chest smoothly and easily.

You may not find this an easy exercise, but persevere. Some students find difficulty because they have allowed the shoulder blades to come apart. To correct this, concentrate awhile on keeping the shoulder blades close together without hollowing the back, and when you feel that you cannot hold the breath longer, draw in the abdomen a little, while relaxing more and more. This will enable you, with a little practice, to finish the count while the breath is held out. But **never strain**. If you cannot, with a little determination, hold the breath out comfortably for more than 10 seconds, be content for a few days to increase gradually. Soon you will manage the count of 20 with ease.

Now try this exercise again in the light of your first effort. Remember, shoulders well back, chest out; and you will breathe correctly, improve your carriage, and, incidentally, help to reduce any tendency to corpulence.

Keeping it up

To obtain the greatest benefit from any form of physical training, correct breathing is absolutely necessary. By physical training, certain muscles are developed at the expense of other parts of the

14

body, and exercise must be regular if the body is not to revert to its former condition. The same is true of massage. Unless you keep it up, the results do not last. Correct breathing should be practiced, continuously until it becomes a habit. As we have seen, it purifies and strengthens the blood, and tones up the muscles which remain ever fresh, "alert", and ready for use.

The athlete, in spite of all his muscular development often has a variety of organic troubles, and is not always the brainiest individual, nor the best example of endurance. Neither is it the strength of muscles alone that raises weights and performs feats of endurance, but the life force resulting from the power of breath.

Summary of Exercise 5

Remind yourself then of this great power of breath as you carry out the exercise. Remember the routine: posture, especially the shoulder blades together, the chin drawn slightly in and down, tongue relaxed, eyes on the concentration spot (this, by the way, also strengthens the accommodative muscles of the eyes).

First the cleansing breath **IN-OUT**, in-out, nine times. Then, without altering the set of the chest, breathe a long **OUT**. Pause: then slowly, fully, fill the lungs. Feel them filling all around—low down, in the front, and in the apices. Next, remembering the puffing engine, breathe **OUT**, out, out, out, out, out, out, out, out; whistle (do not alter the posture). As the whistle dies away, hold the breath and mentally count, one, two, three, four, five, six, seven, eight, nine, ten. Without gasping, breathe **IN** fully, gently and freely. When reaching the top of the inward breath, remember to keep the shoulder steady, blades close together, and breathe **OUT**, out, out, out, out, out, out, out, out; whistle steadily (be careful not to take a breath accidentally) as the remainder of the spent air goes out. Then hold the breath and count, one, two, three, four, five, six, seven, eight, nine, ten, eleven, twelve, thirteen, fourteen, fifteen. Keep control, and breathe **IN**. A long, slow, full breath. You will feel the effect soon enough. You will "feel good". As you progress you will feel better—more vital, and with greater power of mind and body.

Once again breathe **OUT**, out, out, out, out, out, out, out, out; whistle; hold. Concentrate on keeping relaxed, and the muscles controlled, while you count up to 20 seconds.

You are now making the lungs use their full capacity while keeping the pressure of the rib-cage off the lungs and allowing the breathing muscles free play. The lungs now have no alternative; **they**

must breathe to the full. The greater supply of oxygen causes the nerves to relax, with resulting calm.

The whole body, nerves and glands are revived within a few minutes. The knowledge that this can be done should give you feelings of confidence and courage.

Thus, day by day, you will lay a foundation upon which you can build good health, long life, clear mind, greater brain power—all of which make life more worth living,

N.B. Each exercise in this course is to be practiced for **THREE MINUTES**—at least **THREE TIMES A DAY.**

Order of practice

All earlier exercises are to be discontinued until otherwise instructed, with the exception of the cleansing breath and No. 3 which is to be used immediately before the exercise given in this lesson. Thus, two exercises only are to be performed at a time—three times daily.

Powers of Mind are Developed

Postal Course: **LESSON FOUR**

Concentrate on the nose

Many people when doing breathing exercises, try to concentrate their minds on various parts of the body, such as the abdomen or chest. I want you never to concentrate on any part of your body during the exercises except the nose. Whenever you are breathing consciously, as in the exercises, think only of your nose and the air going down or up your windpipe through your nose. Never concentrate on the chest or abdomen as this causes you to make conscious or semi-conscious muscular movements in those regions. This is quite wrong. You must let Nature do the necessary muscle movements on her own, once you have assured the correct body posture. Just concentrate on the nose, and Nature will see that the rest of your breathing apparatus does its job. As you progress with the exercises, the necessary adjustments and improvements in your body are brought about quietly, easily and unconsciously. So, only concentrate on the nose when doing the breathing exercises. This rule, of course, has nothing to do with relaxing (when you do focus your mind on parts of your body in order to relax them).

What to do in stuffy rooms and crowds

Students often ask me if it is not better to breathe as lightly and shallowly as possible when they are in crowded rooms, parties and meetings, or on other occasions when the air is stuffy and smelly. The answer is no: whatever the atmosphere, the slower deeper breathing is always better. However unpleasant the atmosphere seems to be at these times, there is nothing in it which is particularly harmful to the lungs. Its chief characteristic is an increase of carbon dioxide and decrease in oxygen, caused by so many people breathing in poorly-ventilated surroundings. This means that you should be breathing more fully and deeply to take in enough oxygen to give to the blood, as the atmosphere is somewhat "used up". You will of course take in more carbon dioxide as well; but that cannot be put back into your blood via the lungs. The main thing is to extract, out of the poor air, as much oxygen as you can, and breathe out the waste carbon dioxide. Don't bother about the smells in the atmosphere: they won't harm your lungs.

The more you practice correct breathing, the better you will be able to determine the effects upon body and mind. As no doubt you

17

are aware, breath is utilized advantageously by singers, artists and other workers in many fields.

The various functions of breath

Think for a moment of the "outside" functions of breath. Breathe over a dish of hot water, and you will cool it. Breathe into your own cold hands, and you will warm them. Breathe with the outgoing breath softly upon your hand: the result is a gentle warmth. Breathe with the next outgoing breath, again upon your hand but this time mouthing the syllable "pooh", and you will get the opposite result—a gentle, cooling breeze. In this experiment, it does not matter whether you breathe softly, or with increasing force; sometimes another sound may be made, such as "ph" or "f". If you breathe upon your hand gently, and immediately afterwards puff (as in the cleansing breath) you will notice a marked difference.

When you are warm and take in a long breath through your nostrils, exhaling afterwards with lips parted, you get cooled off at once. If, however, you breathe in and out rapidly; then lengthen the breath and continue to alternate; you will start perspiring in a few minutes.

You will already have had enough experience to know that the "it-doesn't-matter-how-you-breathe" school of thought is hopelessly wrong. If you learn to breathe properly, you will master the mind and the body.

Your age, appearance, environment, and the conditions surrounding you do not matter; there is help for all—at all ages and at all times—in the proper use of Breath.

To remind you again that breath is life

Life is completely dependent upon Breath: all forms of Life can only survive by breathing. All animal life has to breathe in order to live: and all plant life has to breathe to live. Oxygen must be continuously absorbed by the cells of body and plant, otherwise they die. If, with the aid of a microscope, we were to look for the germ which constitutes what is commonly called "Life", we should be unable to find it. The microscope would reveal only forms. Nothing could be seen of Breath, the one essential for maintaining Life. We cannot say Life is Breath, any more than we can say that Love is God. The perfect philosopher would say, "God is Love". We consider God to be the Principle of Love as Breath is the Principle of Life. In these lessons you have the opportunity to prove to yourself by your own experience that Breath is Life; and that, by cultivating your breathing powers, you can develop a fuller, richer, healthier, and more harmonious life.

EXERCISE 6. "Recharging" the Nerves by Holding the Breath.

This sixth exercise is one in which you help train the lungs to accept the "idea" or feel, of a breath that permeates the whole lung structure from top to bottom. You will hold this all-pervading breath while the new air is thoroughly mixed with the residual air already in the lungs, and the oxygen is being extracted from this large new supply of in-coming air and given to the blood. It will be found of particular importance in feeding and strengthening the nerve cells, which depend on oxygen for their existence.

Part of the purpose of this exercise is to stimulate and to strengthen the mental controls of the body and brain. You will remember it has already been said that our breathing exercises affect both body and mind. We are now going to breathe IN to the count of 14 seconds (i.e. twice the count of the "key" breath of 7); then to hold the breath (without inducing the slightest strain) while we count 20 seconds; then pause a little, and breathe OUT to the utmost; pause, and breathe IN again for 14 seconds; then pause and count 25 seconds. Again breathe IN twice 7 seconds; pause; hold the breath and count 30 seconds; pause, and breath OUT. Don't forget to concentrate **only on your nose**, as you breathe in and out.

Now for the exercise in detail: take the correct **Posture**, checking over all the details carefully, then thoroughly **Relax**. Take your time to do this; go over and "think into" all the body, legs, arms and head. Then do one or both of the cleansing breaths, the "wood-sawing" one, and the semi-silent whistle-out.

Remember that you are going to breathe in for a longer time. So go gently, and evenly, and **slowly**, us you begin to breathe in.

Now breathe **IN—one** and **two** and **three** and **four** and **five** and **six** and **seven** and **one** and **two** and **three** and **four** and **five** and **six** and **seven** and hold while you count up to 20 seconds; then breathe **OUT** as fully as you can; (without letting go your body posture) pause; and breathe **IN—one** and **two** and **three** and **four** and **five** and **six** and **seven**; and **one** and **two** and **three** and **four** and **five** and **six** and **seven**, and hold to a count of 25 seconds; then breathe **OUT** (keeping shoulder blades in position); pause; breathe **IN—one** and **two** and **three** and **four** and **five** and **six** and **seven** and **one** and **two** and **three** and **four** and **five** and **six** and **seven**, and hold to a count of 30 seconds; pause; then breathe **OUT**.

Repeat this entire exercise three times daily—morning, noon and evening, before meals. If that is not possible, then morning and evening, before meals, and again on retiring for the night.

Of course, 30 seconds held at the end of the in-breath is not the limit of this exercise, but each student must practice according to his or her capacity. **Never strain.** If at first you cannot manage to hold for more than 20 seconds without strain, then repeat this count three times before you can comfortably increase in.

Improvement of the memory

Many people find it hard to believe that, breathing can improve the memory. But it can, as you will find for yourself. It is still one of Nature's mysteries, but I have found in actual practice that holding the breath improves the memory. A good memory involves vividness of impression, strength of retention, and ease of recall. Even if the first two have been attained we often fail to recall quickly and accurately. Whenever a student, through tension or panic, cannot recall a point in an examination, he should breathe **IN** fully; hold the breath for 10 seconds; and breathe **OUT**. Repeat twice. These three breaths held for 10 seconds each will stimulate the mechanism of recall in the brain. Many instances have been recorded in schools and colleges by students who practice this exercise.

Again, if you wish to concentrate deeply and steadily on any subject, you will find great help in the knowledge that calm, deep thought is aided by a full, controlled breath. Test it for yourself. If you are inclined to be nervous and excitable; if you find it difficult to fix your mind on any subject for long; if you read and discover you have not grasped the meaning; **STOP!** Use your breathing exercises. You will quickly experience a steadying of the mind. As this becomes habitual by correct breathing habits, your power of thought, and even your ability to act rightly in emergencies will improve.

The development of brain power and activity depends directly upon the healthy development of your brain cells. Only correct breathing can promote that development, and enable you to grow to your full mental stature.

The four primary breaths

In concluding this lesson, we give the four primary breaths:
1. **BREATHE OUT** for cleansing the lungs.
2. **BREATHE IN** for new oxygen and new life.
3. **HOLD** the breath **OUT** for physical restoration of blood, nerves and glands.

4. **HOLD** the breath **IN** for mental clarity and development of memory.

By the use and control of the breath, you will be able to meet the difficulties and problems of daily experience and health in a new spirit of creative power.

N.B. Each exercise in this course is to be practiced for **THREE MINUTES—THREE TIMES A DAY.**

Order of practice

All earlier exercises are to be discontinued until otherwise instructed, with the exception of No. 3, which is to be used immediately before the exercise given in this lecture, and the cleansing breath. Thus, two exercises only are to be performed at a time—three times daily.

I am starting this lesson with a reminder about **FAITH** not religious faith, but just **FAITH**. A well-known London consultant recently said that all cures of bodily or mental ills could involve anything from about five to twenty percent faith, or belief by the patient that he would get well. That is an amazing statement from a physician, but it is only saying openly what many people have said for centuries. Every hospital nurse will tell you of patients who should, by all the signs, have died; but who have had faith in living, and survived. And of other patients with ordinarily curable complaints who have had no faith, or no particular interest in living, and who have died. This all-parading, but still mysterious "psychosomatic" (mind-body) dependence, means in straight realistic terms that the men or women who have faith in what they are doing, or being done, for them, actually command chemicals to work curatively in their bodies, **irrespective of any medical therapy**. Whereas there is little or no curative chemical link-up in the men and women who have no faith: they must rely entirely on medical therapy, and they often hinder it. If the bodily harm is too great, the former, of course, will die: but the bodily harm can be drastically reduced. If the treatment of the latter can overcome the disease on its own, they will live. But if there is faith, and if the treatment is good, there is a doubly powerful force working for health, working matter-of-factly through the chemicals of the body. What these chemicals are, or exactly how they work, nobody yet knows. But they are present in the body, and faith makes them work. So, when you are living, and breathing, have faith in what you are doing and in the results to be obtained. It will make good results better, and will make them come quicker.

The Power of Faith

How to increase physical fitness and revitalize your body

In all your exercising you should remember two things: first, to concentrate calmly and surely on what you are doing; second, not to overdo any exercise. The moment you feel any sense of strain, check yourself. If you take the correct body posture, with the spinal column erect, and mind set upon the work, effort is no longer needed. You are placed in an attitude of quiet determination and self-reliance that will aid you in gaining the desired effect. The moment you take up your position, however tired you may be, relief comes with the first indrawn breath. After three minutes breathing you will begin to feel refreshed. When you feel tired, exhausted, weary or troubled, do not encourage such conditions to continue through a negative attitude of inertia: rouse yourself and take your breathing exercises.

Breathe into your lungs the centralizing life force which is the ever-acting, never-ending, all-permeating Life Principle, and you will quickly realize your latent powers. With every outgoing breath you part with the forces which have done their work and desire to be liberated into space-forces that are no longer of use to you and from which your heart and lungs need to be cleansed. To retain these forces is harmful to you. These are metaphorical descriptions of the combined action of body, mind and spirit. But they are real enough, and will manifest themselves to anyone whose head is not stuck fast in the sand.

Rest and repose in breath

True rest and repose depend upon correct breathing. Without it, activity is rife, whether you are conscious or unconscious, asleep or awake. When you become restless in sleep, it is often because the lungs are retaining too much carbon and other waste matter that should be set free. If your restlessness awakens you, first breathe the cleansing breath; then slowly fill the lungs; pause; slowly exhale; then pause. Do this twelve times . . and gradually . . . you will . . . drop . . . off . . . to . . . sleep.

Applying the power of breath to digestion, assimilation and excretion

Having now learned how to develop your breath, the time has come when you can apply the new power to both your mental and your physical life. The next exercise applies the power of breath to digestion, assimilation and excretion, by improving the force on which all these depend—the peristaltic action.

Peristaltic Action means the "caterpillar" motion of the intestines (bowels) whereby the food, and later the excreta, is passed through them. If this squeezing motion is not strong or vigorous enough, all the vital processes are slowed down, and ill-health is the inevitable result.

Digestion is the process by which food is used as fuel for the body. Digestion is therefore one of the most important physical functions.

Assimilation is a term little understood by the average person. It means that when the nutriment has been extracted by the digestive system from the food eaten, the elements are passed on to the tissue of cells which constitute our body. These elements are stored up to provide the basic energy which gives us the power of mental and physical action. Few people have good assimilation, and stronger peristaltic action is the remedy.

Excretion is the process of passing out from the body all those parts of the food from which the nutriment has been extracted: it is the waste material for which we have no further use. A healthy person should have one, if not two, bowel excretions daily. If this does not occur, it is because the peristaltic action has become sluggish and inactive. Slowness and dullness of mind are amongst the effects of this condition.

EXERCISE 7. It is now our object to quicken and strengthen these activities by applying the power of correct breathing. This exercise is to be taken three times each day, and may be done **after** meals.

Stand erect with the arms at the side of the body; head up; chin drawn in slightly; eyes steadily gazing upon a concentration spot. The body must be in a calmly relaxed condition, but the spinal column must be firm and erect. The weight of the body should be balanced upon the balls of the feet. No weight should be allowed to rest on the heels. Keep the mouth closed, the teeth separated and the tip of the tongue resting against the lower teeth, as in the first exercise (see illustration A).

After you have taken one of the cleansing breaths, and thoroughly cleared the lungs, breathe **IN** gradually and gently; at the same time swing the right arm (which is to be in a perfectly relaxed condition), with a circular motion in front of you, palm of the hand turned towards the body. Make a perfect circular movement; breathe **IN** while making six circles; breathe **OUT** while making six more circles. Always swing the arm **towards** the body.

After you have swung the right arm round twelve times, bring it up as though to make one more revolution, but **STOP** when the hand is above the head. Clench the fist while taking **IN** a short, quick breath; then, by bending forward with a hip movement and without bending the knees, touch the floor in front of you with the knuckles of the fist. Then rise, at the same time gradually breathe **OUT**, and throw the arm up into the original position, allowing it to drop to the side with a backward circular movement.

Go through the same procedure with the left arm, swinging twelve times as before to a circular motion towards the body; then, as you swing up for the twelfth time, clench the fist, breathe **IN** and touch the floor in front of you as you did with the right arm. (See illustration B.)

Special points to watch in this exercise

Be careful to breathe IN and OUT with a good rhythm. Think of swinging the arm twelve times, and **suit the breath to the swing**. That is to say, you breathe IN while you are making the first six swings, and breathe OUT while you make the second six swings. Keep the swinging going rhythmically. Be particular to hold the breath while making the downward movement to touch the floor, and breathe OUT when bringing the arm back into position.

If you cannot touch the floor at first, do not feel discouraged. Bend the body forward as far as you are able, but **do not bend the knees:** it should be entirely a hip movement.

Don't forget that the hand is to be turned palm **towards** the body, and that the arm is always to be swung parallel with and towards the body. The arm must swing by its own weight perfectly relaxed, and when you drop the hand to the side, let the arm fall and swing until it comes to rest at the side by its own weight.

The Exercise may be taken **after** meals.

Benefits of the exercise

It will aid the digestion. You will find that if a meal has been a trifle too heavy, any tendency to indigestion or dyspepsia will be relieved. In a school where this exercise was practiced, the staff found that it corrected the after-effects of heavy mid-day meals which had often made their pupils sleepy during the afternoon.

Your taste and sense of smell, too, will become more sensitive.

The tendency to constipation is corrected. Children and old people benefit in this respect especially.

Above all, it induces a feeling of buoyancy instead of heaviness, after meals. Teachers and others who have to do evening work will also find the exercise of particular benefit.

So, by attending to the needs of the body, and giving the organs the necessary attention by these exercises and movements, you will vitalize them because you relax the muscles and give the nervous system a greater range of freedom in which to generate its forces. The result will be an improvement in your powers of Digestion, Assimilation and Excretion, and the body will be trained to obey your will.

Breath and the internal organs

Quite apart from the benefits already noted, which correct breathing bring about, there are other important dividends which it pays to those who practice it. One of the fundamental and vital results of the Knowles' System of Breath Training is the training of the diaphragm to flatten (and hence lower) as far as possible, with the simultaneous development of the intercostal muscles, in order to stretch the lungs fully and achieve proper aeration. Now the greater lowering of the diaphragm acts as a valuable massaging device for the abdominal viscera, especially the bowels, both day and night. This lowering of the diaphragm also has a valuable action on the heart, (which rests on the diaphragm); for its pumping action is increased, and this especially helps the venous blood on the final stage of its travel back to the heart. Middle-aged and older people benefit particularly from this, and it is possible that those with a tendency to thrombosis get added relief.

Breath and its exercise provides the way, first to health of body; then to power of mind, and stability of morale. He who would attain true success in life must be able to command and use all three. Nature offers no favors. When we obey her laws, she becomes our willing servant, helping us to be healthy, happy and wise.

N.B. Each exercise in this course is to be practiced for **THREE MINUTES-THREE TIMES A DAY**.

Order of practice

Practice of this 7th exercise is better **after** meals: therefore 3 should be done separately **before** meals three times daily.

Personality and Breath Training

Postal Course: **LESSON SIX**

If you have regularly practiced the exercises given in earlier lessons you should, by now, be conscious that you are more resolute, that your nerves are steadier, your thoughts not so scattered and that you concentrate more easily Whether you have as yet obtained the fullest benefit depends upon the regularity with which you have practiced. So please remember that three things are necessary to acquire and retain the technique of Correct Breathing – **CONCENTRATION – PERSEVERANCE – REGULARITY.**

Morale and the higher forces

This final lesson is a difficult one to write because it concerns forces which are not the measurable and definable forces of science, but forces which many generations of great men have acknowledged, and which most of us feel within us although unable to describe them, and say they are linked with the force of breath. I know that my words will seem to many to be pure metaphysics and symbolism: but if they prove of help even to a few, they are not wasted, if these forces are ever shown to be related to the known forces of science, they will probably be linked with electricity and magnetism.

The first force I will call the Vital Force (the French *élan vital*); the second, the Magnetic Force.

The Vital Force may be symbolized by saying it is enhanced by breath working through the brain: it is the outgoing force of personal power and initiative of creative mind, that influences others, and carries the personality to achievement.

The Magnetic Force may be thought of as working through the heart: it is the center of personal warmth and attraction. The Vital Force at its finest is clear, purposeful and dynamic. The Magnetic Force is sympathetic, attractive and courageous. It is a poor man or woman who develops one at the expense of the other, or who would attempt to belittle either of them.

The science of breath, still so little understood in its higher significance, can help to encourage, develop and unify these two forces, to produce a full and rounded personality. The unifying principle I speak of is also symbolized by the two parts of the breath cycle. The outgoing breath may be seen as gathering together the physical and mental waste products, the negative thoughts and feelings and expelling them from the total personality. The in-drawn breath symbolizes the inspiration of power and positive thinking. The Vital Force and the Magnetic Force each have their waste-products, and their negations. These are combined and expelled, to give way to the life-giving in-breath which flows in to serve both Forces.

As stated at the outset of these lessons, it is the highest aim of the course to lead you into a realization of the fact that your body, your mind and your spirit depend equally for their health, development and harmony upon your breathing. There is only one source, one power, which can perfectly bring about a physical, mental and spiritual balance and unity within you. That source, that power, is breath—the "spiritus" of your being—which brings the Life and Creative Power into your everyday experience. Hold to this truth as the central thought in all your practice. Remember that Breath is Life, and the more fully you breathe, the more abundantly life will be yours.

Remember to relax

In daily work and recreation, and particularly in sport and the various forms of physical training, we are prone to give out our vitality too rapidly. Therefore aim always at relaxing your muscles, using deliberately the power of your imagination in doing so. To strain or to work with hard effort and unrelieved tension is to waste energy and strength. Try to take things calmly, easily and gently. Learn to relax your muscles more and more.

EXERCISE 8. Stand as in the former exercise, bearing in mind that whether standing or walking, you should throw the weight of the body upon the balls of the feet. In other words, **balance** the weight of the body, and you will soon find that there is little weight to the body at all.

As soon as you have taken a cleansing breath, inhale gradually, and throw out your arms in front of you, palms of the hand towards your body, fingers pointing to the ground. Simultaneously cause the muscles to become tensed—not strained. The hands must remain limp at all times: tensing should only occur in the arms and wrists.

In breathing **OUT** relax the muscles again. Repeat, in same position, three times. Three breaths **IN** as you tense from shoulder to wrist: release the muscles as you breathe **OUT**. As you take the fourth breath **IN** tense and move the arms outstretched to the side of the body, even a little to the back—see illustration D. Breathe **OUT**, **IN**, tense-**OUT**, relax, **IN**, tense-**OUT**, relax. As you breathe **IN**, tense (the seventh time), bring the arms back again to position C, with the finger tips facing but not touching. (Illustration E.) **BREATHE OUT** and drop the arms to the side.

At first, you may only notice a peculiar tingling sensation but you may possibly feel a peculiar shock if the fingers touch. This is to be avoided, because the aim is simply to distribute the phosphatic fluids to the extremities of the hands, and later to the extremities of the body generally. This will equalize the electric conditions in the body, and awaken nerve centers which have been inactive. The exercise can be taken three times a day but do not take it more frequently to begin with, nor with more than seven breaths.

EXERCISE 9. Kneel at the back of a chair as in illustration F. bending both knees at the same time. Don't fall on the knees: do it gracefully, as you perform the other exercises. Have the chair at arm's length from you so that you can take hold of the upright bars at the back of the chair, one in each hand. Hands, as well as body, should be perfectly relaxed, and spinal column firm.

After the cleansing breath, breathe **IN** fully and deeply, at the same time tightening your grasp upon the chair bars. Inhale as long as you conveniently can without the use of effort, and without causing any unpleasant feelings in any part of the body—just make yourself quite comfortable. Retain the breath as long as you can with ease, still holding tightly to the chair, and, as you breathe **OUT**, gradually release your hold upon the bars. Exercise in this position for three minutes at a time, and not more than three times a day. You may take the exercise in the evening.

You need not feel concerned if you experience an unusual warmth starting at the navel, and distributing itself over the spinal region in an upward movement to the top of the head as well as downwards to the extremities of the feet. That warmth is caused by the generation of forces in the nervous system, and the cool, fanning sensation which follows it is due to what we might risk calling "magnetic circles".

This exercise rests the mind, producing tranquility and calmness. Therefore you may feel inclined to overdo it. Don't! Like all the other exercises in this course, it is powerful, and the directions for practice should be closely followed.

Remain in the kneeling position, banishing all distracting thoughts from your mind, and follow the current of air as it enters your nostrils, the air tubes and the lungs. As you so relax, your spiritual being will feel its opportunity of development. Even if at first you are not conscious of any special effect, faithful practice will gradually produce within you a physical glow; a feeling of buoyancy; mental illumination, and the sense of an inner spiritual awareness which will uplift you.

The student will notice I have given no names or titles to these last two exercises. I would not know how to describe them. They are based on exercises handed down from oriental antiquity. I have practiced them all my life. Countless thousands of my students have practiced them. I know that my spirit and their spirits have been enhanced and uplifted. We are here beyond the down-to-earth practical results of correct breathing: we are nearing religion. I make no apologies. Those who practice these exercises with humility and faith will benefit vastly: that is all I can say.

The way we have travelled

Thus, step by step, in this course, you have developed your breath capacity; established your lengthened breath, having stepped out of the limitation of your "Mother Breath".

You have trained the sub-conscious side of your being through the strengthening of the sympathetic nerve centers. You have strengthened the **OUT**-breathing technique, ridding the system of excess of carbon dioxide and making the blood better able to resist disease. You have also strengthened the **IN**-breathing technique, and recharged the mental controls through the nervous system, developing your powers of memory and concentration.

Having developed your capacity and use of breath, this newly-acquired power has been directed towards the improvement of your digestion, assimilation and excretion, strengthening the peristaltic action upon which all three depend.

You have developed a new feeling of well-being; a new strength of body and mind to resist disease; and a new method with which to combat disease if it strikes. You have at your command a new technique for curing many ills, especially those that beset the nose, throat and lungs.

Finally, you have within your grasp the ability to develop those higher powers which lie, often dormant, in all of us; powers which transcend body and time and space.

Do not content yourself with merely completing the course

Correct breathing must be practiced until it becomes one of the good habits of your life. This course has shown you how to do that, and by now you should be on the high road to better health and increased vitality.

Continue to breathe correctly throughout your life, and from now onwards you will continue to breathe your way to good health.

Order of practice

For the first week, use Exercise 3 as hitherto, followed by 8 given in this lecture—three times daily. For the second week, use 3 followed by 9—three times daily.

Rota of exercises for future practice

With Lesson 6 you will receive a Rota of Exercises for a further six weeks' practice. The exercises will be precisely as given in this course, but the order will be varied.

COMMON FAULTS

It is but natural that among the thousands of reports from students certain faults and difficulties occur frequently. The Principal therefore thinks it advisable to state some of these common faults and the way to avoid or overcome them.

1. When taking up the posture, be sure you do so simply and easily without any effort. Just gently straighten the spine, tilt forward slightly from the waist and gently draw the shoulder blades as near together as possible, without strain. This should be an effortless poise.

2. The "Cleansing Breath". This is frequently done with far too much vigor. It should be a shallow, gentle breath—like the rhythm of sawing wood.

3. Don't breathe vigorously; just gently and slowly. This applies to all exercises.

4. Don't breathe in and out too quickly. Be sure, when you commence to inhale, that you do so gently and slowly. The same when exhaling; don't allow the breath to escape too quickly.

5. Avoid any abdominal pressure at the end of the exhalation and beginning of inhalation; this can easily be assured by seeing that the shoulders are kept in the correct position.

6. Never use force. Always content yourself with the length of breathing—count you can do with ease; and then gradually extend the count.

7. Don't worry about relaxation. This will follow subconsciously (autonomously) if the simple instructions are carried out.

8. A word to those who suffer from catarrh, asthma, bronchitis or emphysema. Don't be put off by any difficulty in the early stages of the course; patience and perseverance are needed to train the subconscious (sympathetic) nervous system to relax and bring results. What at first may seem almost impossible, will soon become easy with a few weeks of consistent practice, together with calmness, courage and confidence.

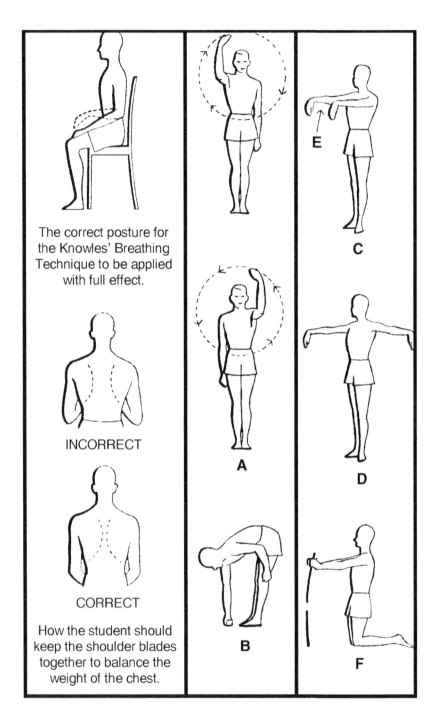

The correct posture for the Knowles' Breathing Technique to be applied with full effect.

INCORRECT

CORRECT

How the student should keep the shoulder blades together to balance the weight of the chest.

E

C

A

D

B

F

THE INSTITUTE OF BREATHING POSTAL COURSE

The value of the Postal Course depends upon continuing the exercises regularly. The following Six Weeks' ROTA OF EXERCISES is for your future guidance and practice.

1st week: SEVEN-SECOND BREATH (Exercise 3, Lesson 2)
EXHALATION (Exercise 4, Lesson 2)

2nd week: SEVEN-SECOND BREATH (Exercise 3, Lesson 2)
INSPIRATION (Exercise 5, Lesson 3)

3rd week: SEVEN-SECOND BREATH (Exercise 3, Lesson 2)
NERVE RECHARGE (Exercise 6, Lesson 4)

4th week: SEVEN-SECOND BREATH (Exercise 3, Lesson 2)
PERISTALTIC (Exercise 7, Lesson. 5)

5th week: SEVEN-SECOND BREATH (Exercise 3, Lesson 2)
VITAL FORCE (Exercise 8, Lesson 6)

6th week: SEVEN-SECOND BREATH (Exercise 3, Lesson 2)
MAGNETIC FORCE (Exercise 9, Lesson 6)

N.B. Each couple of exercises to be practiced three times daily. Three Minutes (not more) to be given to each separate exercise.

34

Printed in Great Britain
by Amazon

82390103R00031